The Keto Diet Cookbook for Beginners

50 Simple Recipes, Weight Loss, Low Carb,
Regain Your Energy

by

SARAH SHELBY

Legal & Disclaimer

Disclaimer and Terms of Use: Effort has been made to ensure that the information in this book is accurate and complete, however, the author and the publisher do not warrant the accuracy of the information, text and graphics contained within the book due to the rapidly changing nature of science, research, known and unknown facts and internet. The Author and the publisher do not hold any responsibility for errors, omissions or contrary interpretation of the subject matter herein. This book is presented solely for motivational and informational purposes only.

The content and information contained in this book has been compiled from sources deemed reliable, and it is accurate to the best of the Author's knowledge, information and belief. However, the Author cannot guarantee its accuracy and validity and cannot be held liable for any errors and/or omissions. Further, changes are periodically made to this book as and when needed. Where appropriate and/or necessary, you must consult a professional (including but not limited to your doctor, attorney, financial advisor or such other professional advisor) before using any of the suggested remedies, techniques, or information in this book.

Upon using the contents and information contained in this book, you agree to hold harmless the Author from and against any damages, costs, and expenses, including any legal fees potentially resulting from the application of any of the information provided by this book. This disclaimer applies to any loss, damages or injury caused by the use and application, whether directly or indirectly, of any advice or information presented, whether for breach of contract, tort, negligence, personal injury, criminal intent, or under any other cause of action.

You agree to accept all risks of using the information presented inside this book.

You agree that by continuing to read this book, where appropriate and/or necessary, you shall consult a professional (including but not limited to your doctor, attorney, or financial advisor or such other advisor as needed) before using any of the suggested remedies, techniques, or information in this book.

Table of Contents

Introduction

I am thank you for purchasing this book, *"The Keto Diet Cookbook for Beginners: 51 Simple Recipes, Weight Loss, Low Carb, Regain Your Energy"*. I hope that this book will help you improve your health and reduce excess weight.

Fats, carbohydrates, and proteins are the three essential macronutrients responsible for a healthy body. Each of them has its special function to the body organs. For example, fats and carbohydrates are broken down to produce energy that helps in the body's physiological functions. In excess, these macronutrients might cause complications such as obesity and cancer. This occurs when you take more than the recommended amount of the nutrients.

Carbohydrates are the immediate sources of energy for the body. Excessive intake of sugars would mean the elevated insulin level to help in breaking down the carbohydrate for the production of energy. The fat in the diet is stored in the tissue resulting in the addition of weight.

Managing our diet is one way to enhance our health. The ketogenic diet is an ancient intervention that was used by the medical practitioners to enhance a metabolic state known as ketosis. This involves lipolysis as the primary source of energy. This recipe substitutes the carbohydrate with the fat as the primary source of energy. Because of the fat breakdown, ketones are produced to supply energy to the brain tissues. This causes a massive reduction in the insulin level as well as that of the blood sugar.

For two centuries, the low-carb diet has been helpful in the medical field.

Ketogenic diet differs from the low-carbohydrate diet. This is because the ketogenic diet replaces the neglected carbohydrate with the increased level of fat concentration. A low-carbohydrate recipe does not take into consideration the protein and fat composition.

Ketones are the by-products of restricted carbohydrate. It is important to determine the ketone bodies within your blood. There are home meters that are used to test the blood for the presence of ketones. Nova Max is an example of a company dealing with strip tests used for the determination of the blood ketone level. They are also able to test the blood glucose level.

It is important we consult our healthcare providers to advise us on the foods that comprise the ketogenic diet. Approximately, our keto diet should include 25% protein, 5% carbohydrates, and 70% fats. This will force the body to utilize the fat for energy at the expense of the carbohydrates. This, therefore, calls for our diet to contain the stated proportions.

Therapeutically, this program can be used for the long-term treatments of epilepsy, diabetes and reducing the seizures.

What is The Ketogenic Diet and why it works.

The human body is one of the most complex organisms in the world. Despite so much research and time, we have still not been able to decipher all of its properties. However more and more progress is made with each passing day. Though people are becoming inclined towards ketogenic diet quite recently, medical evidence suggests that it has been used since almost a century.

Before analyzing what ketogenic diet is and how it actually works, let us shed some light on the scientific origin of it. As the name suggests, it based on the biochemical process of our body that we call Ketogenesis. In this process ketone bodies are produced. These are water soluble molecules that our liver produces from fatty acids when we are fasting or have a very low carbohydrate intake.

Ketone bodies are categorized into three main types namely acetoacetate, acetone and beta-hydroxybutyrate. Acetoacetate and beta-hydroxybutyrate provide energy in the absence of glucose or insulin while acetone is a byproduct that is released into the systems of the body.

Ketosis is the process in which our body burns fat at a very fast rate. This is the foundation for ketogenic diet.

As early as in the 1920s, ketogenic diet was used to help treat epilepsy. As we all know, fasting is an ancient practice that has often been used by people as a way of treating disease. Statistics have revealed that by fasting for eighteen to twenty five days, twenty percent of epileptic patients can be cured while fifty percent would show some improvement.

What is Ketosis you say? Well, it is the natural and healthy metabolic state or process in which the body burns its own stored fat through which it releases a chemical called Ketones which significantly helps to lower down the level of fats in our body and sustain all your activities well. When there is a scarcity of carbohydrate from the food you take, the fat in your body is burnt to provide that energy, which your carbohydrate could not provide. As a consequence of the process, ketones are produced.

An important aspect that you must keep in mind is that you should not get confused between ketosis and ketoacidosis, which is an even more harmful procedure that takes place in the body. However, if you have adequate fat in your body, the ketones are not made use of.

Most importantly, a balanced diet is the best way to have a great metabolism as the optimum amount of fat is burnt and also whether the ketones will be burnt or not is regulated. And if a diabetic with untreated diabetes has ketosis, it is a sign that the hormone insulin is not being optimally utilized in the body.

So, the primary aim of a Ketogenic Diet is to basically down your carbohydrate input to a basal and minimal level, while at the same time doubling on your fat intake.

And this is precisely why Ketogenic Diet has also been known as a High-Fat-Low-carb Diet all around the world.

Thanks to that, Ketogenic Diet is also called "High-Fat-Low-Carb Diet" amongst people of different niche.

Benefits of Ketogenic Diet.

1. Reduced appetite

Ketosis causes lower levels of hunger. You will not feel the need to eat as much as you previously did.

2. Low levels of cholesterol

Ketogenic diet increases the "good cholesterol and HDL". As glucose intake is diminished, your overall cholesterol level would be controlled. This is important for your long term health as cholesterol tends to accumulate in veins and lead to problems like stroke, heart diseases, high blood pressure etc.

3. Lesser chance of hypertension

The reduced intake of carbohydrates results in lower blood pressure. This again prevents against other diseases too which include heart disease, depression and damage to vital organs of the body.

4. Avoiding hypogycemia

As your body becomes less reliant on sugar and glucose, the craving for foods with these ingredients is reduced. Your body learns to live without adequate sugar in the blood.

5. Reduced triglycerides

Carbohydrates directly affect the level of triglycerides. Low levels of triglycerides reduce the risk of a heart attack.

6. Lesser chance of arthritis

Joint pain, among other things, is also caused by excessive weight. As ketogenic diet allows you to be leaner, chances of developing arthritis are also decreased.

7. Clarity of mind

As we discussed earlier in this chapter, ketogenic diet enhances brain performance and hence allows you to think more clearly.

8. Better digestion

Although some patients complain of constipation in the initial days of ketogenic diet, if combined with the right amount of fluids and fiber it actually helps make the digestion process more efficient. Your metabolism is improved steadily.

9. Mood stability

Again, the experiments regarding mood with the users of this diet have provided conflicting results. However, it is sometimes suggested that as you feel fitter, it actually puts you in a better mood.

10. Better dental health

Sugar causes tooth decay and gum problems. With ketosis this can easily be avoided.

11. Relief from heartburn

With a healthier blood composition, heartburn can be reduced if not completely eliminated. Ketogenic diet removes foods, which induce heartburn, from your life which include sugary foods, grains etc.

12. Greater physicall fitness

The reduced weight helps you to be lighter on your feet and has many cosmetic as well as medical benefits.

12. Better sleep

Ketogenic diet has shown a better sleeping pattern in people. This is because your metabolism and this soothes your body.

13. Fights cancer

As we all know, cancer feeds off sugar in the body. With ketosis, the prevention against this deadly disease rises.

14. More energy

Despite initial complains of fatigue, the diet makes you much more active and productive.

What we eat and what we don't.

What To Eat

To make everything simple, remind yourself while shopping that you want to eat real food. Of course, your main objective is to cut out and limit your carbohydrate intake. As you do this, try your best to avoid foods that contain colorings, preservatives and have been processed. To make it easy, we will provide you with a list of foods you can consume and foods you should rather eat moderately. Then we will provide you with a list of foods you should avoid altogether. Finally, check out our last chapter for delicious recipes to show you that a diet never needs to be bland!

Eat a Majority of These:

Meat, including lamb, goat, venison, or beef; Fish & seafood (wild when possible); Poultry and pork; Beef; Bacon; Eggs; Butter; Ghee; Gelatin; Kidneys, liver, heart, and other grass-fed organs; Mayonnaise; Pesto; Bone broth; Mustard; Pork rinds; Coffee; Herbal tea; WATER

Vegetables - Non-Starchy; Celery; Cucumber; Zucchini; Summer squash; Shoots of bamboo; Asparagus; Kale; Radishes; Kohlrabi; Chives; Chard; Bok choy; Swiss chard; Radicchio; Any other leafy greens; Healthy Fats.

Spices: Cumin; Parsley; Rosemary; Sage; Cinnamon; Cilantro; Cayenne Pepper; Black Pepper; Sea Salt; Basil; Turmeric; Oregano.

Saturated fats including: duck fat, goose fat, chicken fat, lard, ghee, coconut oil, regular butter.

Polyunsaturated Omega 3s: You can get these from seafood and other fatty fish.

Monosaturated fat, including olive oil, macadamia, avocados.

Healthy Condiments and Beverages: Any spices or herbs are allowed. We suggest using lemon and lime juice to spice up any recipe.

Whey protein. When you choose your protein, be aware of any additives. Many proteins add hormones, soy, and artificial sweeteners.

Eat These In Moderation:

Nuts and Seeds: Pecans; Walnuts; Almonds; Hazelnuts; Flaxseed; Pine nuts; Sesame seeds; Pumpkin seeds; Hemp seeds; Sunflower seeds; Macadamia nuts; Brazil nuts.

Dairy: Plain yogurt; Sour cream; Cheese; Cottage cheese.

Be sure that these are all full fat. Low-fat has added sugar that you do not need.

Grain-fed Animal Protein. Sometimes it can be difficult to get grass-fed protein. In that case, you can eat grain-fed animal protein in moderation. However, try to avoid farmed pork. This specific animal protein will be high in omega 6 fatty acids, which you want to avoid.

Fruits and Vegetables: Root vegetables, including onion, mushrooms, garlic, winter squash, spring onions, leeks, and parsley root; Sea vegetables, including bean sprouts, wax beans, water chestnuts, French artichokes, okra, sugar snap peas; Coconut; Olives; Rhubarb; Eggplant; Peppers; Tomatoes. Cruciferous vegetables, including cabbage, broccoli, fennel, rutabaga, turnips, Brussels sprouts and cauliflower. Berries in moderation, including strawberries, blueberries, cranberries, blackberries and mulberries. Root vegetables (depending on carb limit): celery root, beetroot, sweet potato, parsnip, carrot.

Fruits (depending on carb limit): peach, apple, kiwi, orange, cherries, pears, plums, figs, apricot, nectarine, dragon fruit.

Beverages: Alcohol can be included, in moderation. Be sure to limit it to special occasions to help your weight loss. Dry red wine; Spirits – unsweetened; Dry white wine.

Condiments: Tomato products (sugar-free) including: ketchup, puree, and passata. Cocoa powder: try your best to stick to 90%. Healthy sweeteners, including swerve & stevia. Thickeners, including xanthan gum & arrowroot powder.

Soy: If you want to include soy products in your diet, be sure they are fermented. This way, you know that they do not contain GMOs. Soy sauce; Tempeh; Natto; Edamame; Black soybeans.

What Not To Eat

Grains: Whole meal, including sprouted grains, buckwheat, rye, corn, oats, wheat, bulgur, amaranth, sorghum, white potatoes and quinoa. Other grains, including bread, pasta, crackers, cookies, pizza, etc. Sweets, including puddings, ice cream, agave syrup, soft drinks.

Processed Foods: MSGS: These can be found in whey protein. Carrageenan: These are normally found in almond milk. BPAs. Wheat gluten. Sulphites.

Factory Farmed Foods: Pork- High in Omega 6 Fatty Acids; Fish- May contain PCBs and high levels of mercury.

Milk: If you want to keep milk in your diet, try to limit it to full fat milk in small amounts. This may be a bad idea because milk can be hard to digest for some people. Dairy is also high in carbs. You can substitute milk with cream when needed.

Fruits: Mainly, you will want to avoid tropical fruits. These include banana, mango, pineapple, papaya; High carb fruits, including grape & tangerine; Fruit juices; Dried fruits.

Low-fat: When reading labels, avoid anything low-carb, low-fat, or zero-carb; Diet soda; Chewing gum; Atkins products; Artificial sweeteners, including Equal, Splenda, and anything that includes Aspartame.

Refined Fats & Oils: Corn, canola, cottonseed, sunflower, safflower, soybean and grape seed oil; Anything with trans fats.

Breakfast Recipes

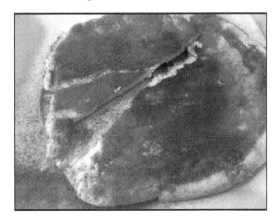

High Protein Mascarpone Pancakes

Preparation time: 5 mins

Servings: 2

Nutritional Information: 546 Calories, 41g Fats, 12g Net Carbs, and 33g Protein.

Ingredients:

- 6 eggs
- 1 c. mascarpone cheese
- ¼ c. ground flax seeds
- ¼ c. chia seeds
- 1½ tsps. baking powder
- Salt

Directions:

1. Combine the flaxseed, chia seeds, baking powder and salt in a bowl. Add the eggs to the dry ingredients one at a time, whisking well after each egg.

2. Add mascarpone cheese and mix until smooth. Alternatively, place all the ingredients in a blender to achieve the same results. If you want to sweeten the batter, add about a teaspoon of sugar substitute at this point and mix well.

3. Spray cooking oil spray on a non-stick skillet and set over medium-high heat.

4. Use a large spoon or, preferably, a ladle to pour the pancake batter into the skillet once the skillet is hot.

5. Let the pancake to cook for approximately 3 minutes before carefully flipping it over with a spatula. Change to the other side and cook for approximately 2 minutes. Adjust the timing accordingly if you would prefer your pancakes more or less browned.

6. Serve pancakes with butter, low-carb syrup, sour cream or berries — or any combination of these options!

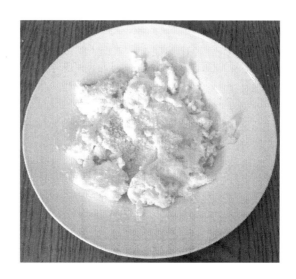

Parmesan Eggs

Preparation time: 4 mins

Servings: 1

Nutritional Information: 308 Calories, 27.2g Fats, 1.9g Net Carbs, and 15.8g Protein.

Ingredients:

- 2 tbsps. Parmesan cheese, fresh and grated
- 1 tbsp. whipping cream
- 1 tbsp. butter, melted
- 1 egg

Directions:

1. Preheat the oven to 350 degrees F.
2. Grease the ramekin with the butter. Dust with 1 tablespoon of the Parmesan cheese.

3. Crack the egg into the ramekin and cover with the cream. Sprinkle the remaining cheese to the mixture; bake for about 10-15 minutes, or until the egg white is set. Serve hot inside the ramekin.

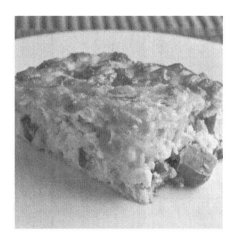

Breakfast Squares

Preparation time: 5 mins

Servings: 3

Nutritional Information: 782 Calories, 62.6g Fats, 4.4g Net Carbs, and 51.6g Protein.

Ingredients:

- 8 ounces mozzarella cheese, shredded
- 8 ounces cheddar cheese, shredded
- 6 large eggs, beaten
- Sliced Jalapeno peppers
- 4 tbsps. butter

Directions:

1. Carefully mix the cheeses and eggs.

2. Butter the bottom of a skillet; add the pepper and the cheese mixture; Set oven to 350F, and bake for 35 minutes, then for 30 more minutes at 250 degrees F.

3. Serve

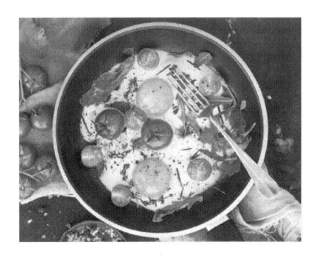

Italian Breakfast

Preparation time: 15 mins

Servings: 2

Nutritional Information: 189 Calories, 3g Fats, 5g Net Carbs, and 7g Protein.

Ingredients:

- 2 eggs
- 4 slices prosciutto ham
- 1 peeled clove organic garlic
- ½ c. rocket lettuce
- 10 halved cherry tomatoes
- Sea salt
- Ground black pepper
- 4 tbsps. butter

Directions:

1. Set your oven to medium-high heat. Place a tablespoon of butter in a small skillet and heat.

2. Crack and fry the eggs, preferably sunny side up, until the edges are golden (usually around 3-4 minutes). Remove from the heat and set the mixture aside for the moment.

3. Next, peel and crush the garlic clove. If need be, add more butter. Add garlic to the skillet and sauté until it begins to turn a golden brown. Add a dash of salt and pepper.

4. Sauté the halved tomatoes for about 2–3 minutes, turning half way.

5. Optionally, saute the rocket and prosciutto for 30 seconds.

6. Everything should be ready to serve, add salt and pepper according to your taste.

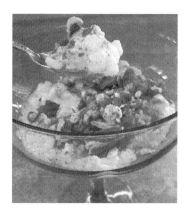

Breakfast Low Carb Mock Cinnamon

Preparation time: 3 minutes

Servings: 1

Nutritional Information: 339 Calories, 28.3g Fats, 7.7g Net Carbs, and 16.6g Protein.

Ingredients:

- ½ c. cottage cheese

- 7 toasted pecan halves

- 1 g stevia

- Cinnamon, ground

- 1½ tbsps. ghee

Directions:

1. In a large bowl, mix ghee, cottage cheese, and the sweetener.

2. Sprinkle with cinnamon and then top with the pecan halves. Serve.

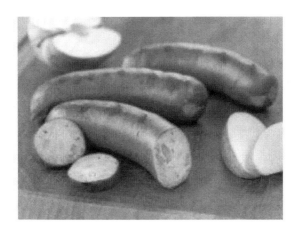

Apple Sausages

Preparation time: 5 mins

Servings: 6

Nutritional Information: 162 Calories, 13.7g Fats, 9.2g Net Carbs, and 2.1g Protein.

Ingredients:

- 2 peeled, cored and diced medium sized apples
- 6 breakfast sausage links
- 4 tbsps. vegetable oil
- 1 tbsp. brown sugar

Directions:

1. Place the links in a cast-iron frying pan. Pour enough water to cover the bottom of the pan. Add the oil.

2. Set oven to medium heat and heat to evaporate water and the sausages start to change to brown.

3. Add the sweetener and apples. Cook, stirring the apple in the sausage grease, until the apples are tender.

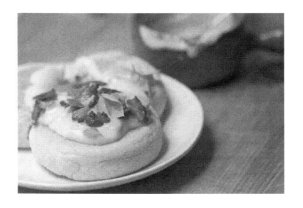

Bacon Gravy

Preparation time: 5 mins

Servings: 4

Nutritional Information: 393 Calories, 35.5g Fats, 13.4g Net Carbs, and 8.9g Protein.

Ingredients:

- 6 slices bacon
- 2 c. almond milk
- 2 tbsps. tapioca flour
- 2 tbsps. bacon grease
- Pepper
- Salt

Directions:

1. Set your oven to medium high and preheat a skillet. Add bacon and cook for some time to make it crispy.

2. Remove the bacon; set aside. Drain the grease, leaving 2 tablespoons in the skillet and saving the rest for other cooking use.

3. To the skillet, add the flour and carefully whisk to combine. Take 1 minute to heat the mixture.

4. Add the milk, whisk to combine, and bring to simmer; cook for about 5-10 minutes or until the sauce starts to thicken.

5. Meanwhile, crumble the bacon. Add pepper and salt to enhance taste. Add the bacon into the gravy. Simmer until you attain a desired consistency. Serve with biscuits.

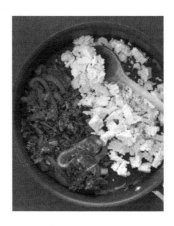

Cajun Tofu Scramble

Preparation time: 13 mins

Servings: 2

Nutritional Information: 224 Calories, 12g Fats, 14g Net Carbs, and 22g Protein.

Ingredients:

- 14 ounces drained and cubed tofu
- ½ yellow onion
- 1 diced red bell pepper
- 1 diced zucchini
- 2 teaspoon Cajun seasoning
- Kale

Directions:

1. Saute onions in a skillet until transparent. Add tofu and seasonings. Cook for five minutes. Add vegetables and cook until tender, approximately eight minutes.

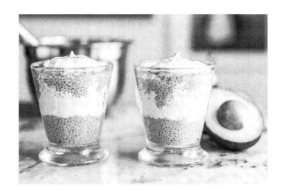

Avocado Chia Seed Pudding

Preparation time: 4 mins

Servings: 4

Nutritional Information: 273 Calories, 24g Fats, 15g Net Carbs, and 4g Protein.

Ingredients:

- ¼ c. chia seeds
- 1 ripe avocado, black-skinned
- 1 c. coconut milk
- 2 medium-sized dates
- ½ teaspoon vanilla extract

Directions:

1. Blend avocado with coconut milk, dates, and spices. Pour mixture over chia seeds. Cover and refrigerate overnight.

Lunch Recipes

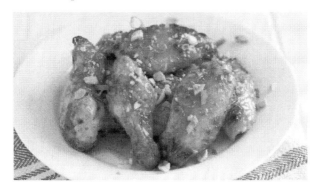

Garlicky Chicken Livers

Preparation time: 5 mins

Servings: 1

Nutritional Information: 858 Calories, 68.3g Fats, 5.1g Net Carbs, and 56.1g Protein.

Ingredients:

- ½ pound chicken liver
- 1 tsp. lemon juice
- 2 tbsps. olive oil
- 2 tbsps. melted ghee
- 3 cloves garlic
- Salt

Directions:

1. Wash the chicken livers. Trim and dry them.

2. Dry-fry them in a nonstick frying pan for about 4 minutes without the use of oil.

3. To the pan, add lemon juice, ghee-olive oil, and salt to taste. Stir once to mix.

4. Sprinkle the garlic and serve.

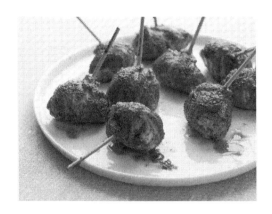

Chicken Bacon Wraps

Preparation Time: 25 minutes

Servings: 12

Nutritional Info: Calories 502, Total Fat 38.2 g, Protein 38.1 g, Total Carbs 1.1 g

Ingredients:

- 12 skinless and boneless chicken breast halves
- 12 slices of bacon
- 16 oz. chive and onion cream cheese
- 12 tbsps. divided olive oil spread
- Salt

Directions:

1. Flatten the chicken breasts to 1/2-inch thickness.

2. Spread 3 tablespoons of cream cheese over each chicken breast.

3. Dot with 1 tablespoon olive oil spread and sprinkle with the salt; roll up and wrap each rolled piece with a bacon strip.

4. Grease your pan and place chicken onto it and bake uncovered for about 40 minutes at 400 degrees F or until the juices run clear.

5. Transfer the pan 6 inches from the heat source; broil for 5 minutes until the bacon is crispy.

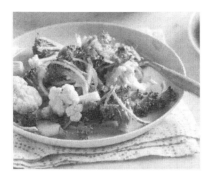

Cauliflower Salad

Preparation time: 10 mins

Servings: 4

Nutritional Info: Calories 588, Total Fat 49 g, Protein 19 g, Total Carbs 19 g

Ingredients:

Salad:

- 1 head cauliflower, medium
- 1½ c. mushrooms, sliced
- 1½ tbsps. olive oil
- 1 tsp. fresh dill
- 1 tsp. chives, chopped
- ½ tsp. paprika, smoked
- Salt
- Pepper

Sauce:

- ½ c. extra-virgin olive oil

- ¼ c. soy milk, unsweetened

- 1 tsp. cider vinegar, raw

- Salt

- White pepper

Directions:

1.   Make the salad; cut cauliflower into tiny florets.

2.   Place the cauliflower florets into a pan and cover with water.

3.   Bring to a boil and reduce heat. Simmer for 3-4 minutes or until crisp tender.

4.   In the meantime, heat olive oil in a skillet. Cook mushrooms for 5-8 minutes or until soft. Toss in the cauliflower and shake to coat with oil. Season to taste with salt and pepper.

5.   Make the sauce; make sure oil and milk are equal temperatures. It is a very important step.

6.   Place soy milk, cider vinegar, and seasonings in a food blender. Blend until smooth. While the blender is running low, gradually stream in extra-virgin olive oil.

7.   Blend until thickens.

8.   In a bowl, toss cauliflower with prepared sauce, dill, and chives.

9.   Divide between bowls and sprinkle with paprika. Chill briefly before serving.

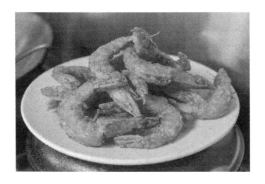

Salt-and-Pepper Stir-Fried Shrimp

Preparation time: 16 mins

Servings: 6

Nutritional Info: Calories 335, Total Fat 10.6 g, Total Carbs 4.8 g, Protein 52 g,

Ingredients:

- 4 cloves garlic, chopped

- 2 tsps. divided salt

- 2 tbsps. vegetable

- 2 pounds shrimp

- Red, white, black, and green peppercorns (½ tsp. each)

- 1 c. chopped cilantro leaves

Directions:

1. Crush the peppercorns in a mortar.

2. Into a large bowl, place the shrimp, salt and half of the crushed peppercorns; toss to coat the shrimp evenly and set aside.

3. Heat a large nonstick pan over high heat. Add the garlic, oil, and the remaining peppercorns and salt; cook for about 1 minute, constantly stirring, until fragrant.

4. Add the shrimp to the mixture and cook for about 4 minutes as you stir.

5. Add the cilantro; turn off the heat; and toss to combine. Serve right away.

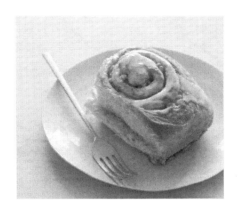

Almond Buns

Preparation Time: 15 mins

Servings: 6

Nutritional Info: Calories 184, Total Fat 17.2 g, Protein 4.7 g, Total Carbs 4.3 g

Ingredients:

- 2 eggs

- ¾ c. almond flour

- 5 tbsps. Butter, unsalted

- 1½ tsp. baking powder

- 1½ tsp. stevia or Splenda

Directions:

1. Combine the dry ingredients in a bowl.

2. Whisk in the eggs.

3. Melt butter and add it to the mixture.

4. Divide the mixture into equal 6 parts; place into a muffin top pan or something similar.

5. Bake at 350 degrees F for about 12-17 minutes. You may need to watch the first time you make these, since cooking time will vary depending on your oven.

6. Let cool on a wire rack.

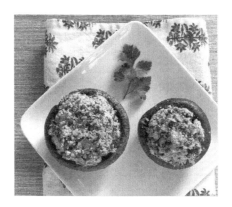

Stuffed Portabella With Nut Pate

Preparation time: 10 mins

Servings: 4

Nutritional Info: Calories 158, Total Fat 9.4 g, Protein 10 g, Total Carbs 12.7 g

Ingredients:

- 4 portabella mushrooms caps
- 1 tbsp. olive oil
- 1 tbsp. coconut aminos
- Pepper
- Salt
- Nut pate:
- 1 c. soaked macadamia nuts
- 1 tbsp. coconut aminos
- 1 chopped celery stalk

- Kosher salt

Directions:

1.   Heat oven to 375F and line a baking sheet with parchment paper.

2.   In a bowl, beat olive oil with coconut aminos. Brush in mushroom caps with oil mixture and arrange onto a baking sheet.

3.   Bake for 15 minutes.

4.   In the meantime, make the nut pate; rinse and drain macadamia nuts. Place the macadamia nuts and celery in a food processor and process until just smooth. In the last seconds of processing, add coconut aminos and salt to taste.

5.   Process until the coconut aminos is incorporated.

6.   Remove the portabella from the oven and place on a plate. Fill with macadamia pate and serve warm.

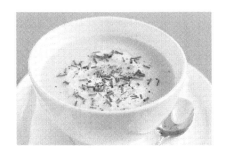

Creamy Cauliflower Soup

Preparation time: 10 mins

Servings: 4

Nutritional Info: Calories 240, Total Fat 1 g, Protein 10 g, Total Carbs 50 g

Ingredients:

- 2 c. cauliflower florets

- 2 c. wild mushrooms, sliced

- 2 c. coconut milk, full-fat

- 2 tbsps. avocado oil

- 1 tsp. celery flakes, dried

- ½ tbsps. Thyme, freshly chopped

- 1 minced clove garlic

- Salt

- Pepper

Directions:

1.   In a saucepan, mix celery flakes, cauliflower, and coconut milk.

2.   Cover and bring to a boil over medium-high heat.

3.   Reduce heat and simmer for 6-7 minutes. Kill the heat and puree using an immersion blender.

4.   In the meantime, heat avocado oil in a skillet. Add thyme and garlic. Cook until fragrant. Toss in wild mushrooms and cook for 6-7 minutes or until tender.

5.   Pour in pureed cauliflower and bring to a boil. Reduce heat and simmer 6-8 minutes or until thickened.

6.   Serve warm with Keto bread.

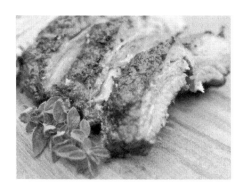

Spicy Garlic Butter Shrimp

Preparation time: 15 mins

Servings: 5

Nutritional Information: 749 Calories, 30.7g Fats, 8.3g Net Carbs, and 103.8 g Protein.

Ingredients:

- 4 pounds large-sized shrimp, unpeeled
- 1 -2 tablespoons garlic, minced
- ½ cup butter
- Lemon pepper seasoning
- Garlic powder

Directions:

1. Preheat the oven to 300 degrees F.
2. Mix the butter and the garlic.
3. Place the shrimp in a saucepan and dot with the garlic butter; sprinkle well with the garlic powder and the lemon pepper.

4. In an uncovered state, bake for about 30 minutes, stirring once or twice, until the shrimp is opaque, making sure the shrimp is evenly cooked.

5. Serve alongside the butter sauce that is in a separate bowl or the one containing the shrimp for dipping.

6. You may serve alongside cauliflower rice.

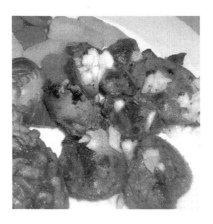

Sticky Drumsticks

Preparation time: 5 mins

Servings: 8

Nutritional Information: 209 Calories, 16.7g Fats, 1.2g Net Carbs, and 13.4g Protein.

Ingredients:

- 8 chicken drumsticks
- ½ c. olive oil
- ¼ c. sweet chili sauce
- 2 garlic cloves, minced
- ¼ c. soy sauce
- 2 tsps. sesame seeds

Directions:

1. Slice through the thickest part of each drumstick using a sharp knife. Arrange them in a glass dish.

2. In a bowl, mix the sauces and garlic. Rub all over the drumstick; marinate for about 30 minutes in the refrigerator.

3. Preheat the oven to 120C of 180 for fan.

4. Place the drumsticks on a nonstick baking paper. Sprinkle them with sesame seeds. Bake for about 45 minutes. Let cool slightly; serve.

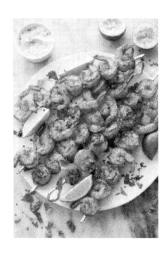

Grilled Spicy Lime Shrimp

Preparation time: 5 mins

Servings: 8

Nutritional Information: 188 Calories, 3g Fats, 1.2g Net Carbs, and 13g Protein.

Ingredients:

- 1 pound peeled and deveined medium shrimp
- 1 juiced lime
- ½ c. vegetable oil
- 3 tbsps. Cajun seasoning

Directions:

1. In a Ziploc bag, mix the Cajun seasoning, lime juice, and vegetable oil. Add the shrimp, shake to coat, squeeze out the excess air, seal the bag, and marinate for 20 minutes in the refrigerator.

2. Preheat an outdoor grill to medium heat. Lightly grease the grate.

3. Take the shrimp from marinade as you shake off any excess; discard marinade.

4. Allow to cook both sides for 2 minutes each. Serve.

Dinner Recipes

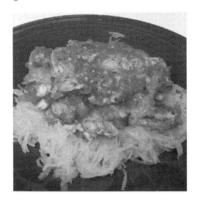

Chicken Cacciatore with Spaghetti Squash

Preparation time: 90 mins

Servings: 6

Nutritional Info: Calories 267, Total Fats 5.1g, Protein 40g, Total Carbs 17g

Ingredients:

- 4 skinless and boneless chicken thighs

- 1 medium diced Onion

- 1 large bell peppers

- 2 minced cloves Garlic

- ½ tsp. thyme, dried

- 1 c. Chicken stock

- 28 oz. tomatoes, diced

- 8 oz. Tomato sauce

- ½ tsp. dried basil

- Salt

- Pepper

- ½ diced yellow squash

- ½ tsp. dried oregano

- 1 Spaghetti squash

Directions:

1. Dice the veggies. Set them aside.

2. Cut the chicken up. Season it as desired.

3. Place the chicken in a Dutch oven and let it brown for about 8 minutes.

4. Add in the onion, garlic and bell pepper and let them cook for approximately 5 minutes or until the onions soften.

5. Add the chicken tomato sauce, tomatoes, and the chicken stock.

6. Season as desired and mix well before letting everything boil.

7. Turn the heat to low and let everything cook for 30 minutes.

8. Add the yellow squash. Cook between 15 and 30 more minutes.

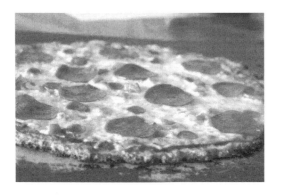

Meat-Based Pizza

Preparation time: 15 mins

Servings: 1

Nutritional Info: Calories 195, Total Fats 24g, Protein 17g, Total Carbs 1.2g

Ingredients:

- Small package of Ground uncooked beef

- Salsa

- 1 diced Onion

- Italian Spices

- Garlic powder

- Shredded Mozzarella cheese

- 6 strips Bacon

Directions:

1. Dice onion and put the onion into a baking dish.

2. Add the beef, salsa, garlic powder and other spices into a baking dish. Mix together.

3. Shred the cheese and put it evenly over the top of the beef mixture.

4. Cut the bacon into small pieces and put the pieces on top of the cheese.

5. Ensure your oven is set to 375 degrees F.

6. Place the pizza in the oven and let it cook for 35 minutes.

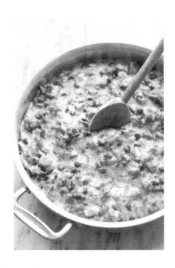

Mexican Casserole

Preparation time: 15 mins

Servings: 12

Nutritional info: Calories 69, Total Fats 30g, Protein 3.56g, Total Carbs 4.5g

Ingredients:

- ½ tsp. Cumin
- 1 head Cauliflower
- ½ white Onion
- ½ tsp. Chili powder
- 1 Green bell pepper
- 1½ c. Parmesan
- 1 hashed Bell pepper
- 4 chopped Cherry tomatoes

Directions:

1. Ensure your oven is set to 350 degrees Fahrenheit.

2. Place the skillet on top of the stove over a burner set to a medium heat.

3. Roast the chili powder, pepper, cumin and onion, stirring regularly until the veggies are fully cooked.

4. Dice the cauliflower. Cook it in the microwave for 3 minutes.

5. Put the tomatoes and 1 cup of the cheese in with the cauliflower. Mix.

6. Mix the results with the vegetables.

7. Using cooking spray coat a baking dish.

8. Add the vegetable mixture to the baking dish.

9. Add the rest of the cheese.

10. Place the dish in the oven and let it cook for approximately 40 minutes.

11. Garnish as desired.

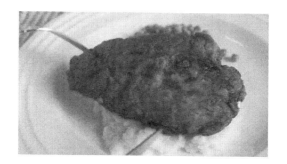

Tasty Fried Chicken Breast

Preparation time: 10 mins

Servings: 1

Nutritional Info: Calories 189, Total Carbs 1g, Protein 27g, Total Fat 8g

Ingredients:

- 1 Chicken breast
- Butter
- Salt
- Pepper
- Curry powder
- Garlic powder
- ½ c. Greens

Directions:

1. Cut chicken into small chunks.
2. Heat up the butter in a frying pan.

3. Put the chicken into the pan. Stir to coat chicken.

4. Add spices to taste.

5. Stir fry until the chicken browns and gets crunchy.

6. Serve with greens on the side.

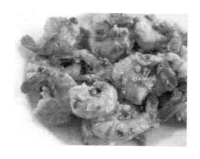

Baby-Back Ribs

Preparation time: 5 mins

Servings: 4

Nutritional Information: 1252 Calories, 81.1g Fats, 3.8g Net Carbs, and 120.7g Protein.

Ingredients:

- 4 pounds baby back pork ribs
- 2 tbsps. sugar
- 2 tbsps. chili powder
- ½ tsp. mustard powder
- ½ tsp. thyme leaves, dried
- Salt

Directions:

1. Preheat the oven to 300F or light an outdoor grill.
2. In a small bowl, except for the ribs, combine the rest of the ingredients; rub the mixture on each side of the ribs.
3. If using a grill, cook the ribs with the bone-side down over medium-low heat or when the coals are covered

with ash. Adjust the flame and add coals if necessary; cook for about 1½ hours.

4. If using an oven, place the ribs with the bone-side down; cook for 1½ hours.

5. The ribs are cooked when the ribs separate when you insert a fork between them.

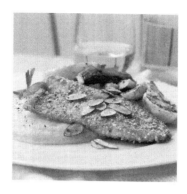

Almond-Crusted Tilapia

Preparation time: 15 mins

Servings: 4

Nutritional Information: 415 Calories, 26.2g Fats, 11.5g Net Carbs, and 36.7g Protein.

Ingredients:

- 4 (each 6 ounces) tilapia fillets

- 2 tbsps. olive oil

- 2 tbsps. butter

- ¼ cup tapioca flour

- Salt

- 1 c. sliced and divided almonds

Directions:

1. Place ½ cup of the almonds in the food processor until chopped into fine pieces. Transfer into a shallow bowl. Add the flour, mix until combined.

2. Evenly sprinkle the fillets with salt and dredge with the almond-flour mixture.

3. In a large skillet, melt the butter with the olive oil over medium heat. Add the fish; cook for about 4 minutes per side or until golden brown. Transfer the fillets into a serving plate.

4. Add the remaining almond into the skillet; cook for 1 minute, frequently stirring, or until golden.

5. With a slotted spoon, remove the almonds; sprinkle over the fillets.

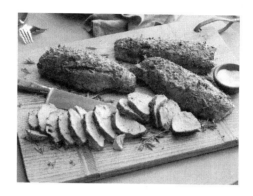

Perfect Boneless Pork Tenderloin

Preparation time: 5 mins

Servings: 4

Nutritional Info: 162 Calories, 4g Fats, 0g Net Carbs, and 29.7g Protein.

Ingredients:

- 1 pound pork tenderloin, boneless

- Onion powder

- Any of the following or a mixture (thyme, rosemary, garlic powder, or savory)

- Salt

- Pepper

Directions:

1. Determine the exact weight of your roast from the meat wrapper. This will determine how long you need to cook it.

2. Preheat the oven to 500F.

3. Season the meat according to your preference. Place uncovered on a shelf in the bottom 1/3 of the oven.

4. Bake EXACTLY for 5½ minutes PER POUND. Adjust the time according to your oven's heat retention and accuracy.

5. Turn the oven off. Do not open the door for about 45 minutes to 1 hour. If your oven has a probe thermometer, you can open the oven door when it alerts that the temperature is 140F.

6. Remove the pork from the oven; cover lightly with foil; and let rest for about 5 -10 minutes to redistribute the internal juices.

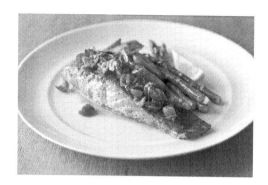

Basil Tomato Salmon

Preparation time: 10 mins

Servings: 2

Nutritional Information: 374 Calories, 41.6g Fats, 1.8g Net Carbs, and 37.9g Protein.

Ingredients:

- 2 boneless salmon fillets
- 4 tbsps. olive oil
- 1 thinly sliced tomato
- 1 tbsp. basil, dried
- 2 tbsps. Parmesan cheese, grated

Directions:

1. Preheat the oven to 375F or 190C.
2. Take an aluminum foil and line the baking sheet and grease it with nonstick cooking spray.

3. Place the salmon on the foil; sprinkle with the basil; top with the tomato; drizzle with the olive oil, or sprinkle with parmesan.

4. Bake for about 20 minutes, or until the salmon center is opaque and the cheese is lightly browned on top.

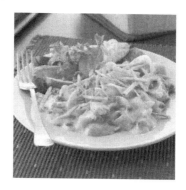

Cheesy Tuna Casserole

Preparation time: 20 mins

Servings: 4

Nutritional Information: 459 Calories, 33g Fats, 12g Net Carbs, and 31g Protein.

Ingredients:

- 12 ounces drained Tuna
- 16 oz. frozen Green beans
- 3 oz. sliced fresh mushrooms
- 2 tbsps. Butter
- ½ c. Chicken broth
- ¾ c. Heavy cream
- 2 chopped Onions
- Salt
- Pepper
- Xanthan gum

- 1 stalk hashed Celery

- 8 oz. shredded Cheddar cheese

Directions:

1. Cook the green beans in a medium pot. Drain well.

2. Place the butter, celery, mushrooms and onion in a pan and place the pan on top of the stove over a burner turned to a medium heat and let everything cook for 5 minutes.

3. Add the broth. Boil, letting the liquid cook down by half.

4. Stir in the cream. Let come back up to a boil.

5. Turn down the heat until the sauce is thickened, stirring frequently. Don't let it boil over.

6. Season to taste.

7. Put the mushroom and tuna mixture into the green beans.

8. Add salt and pepper if needed.

9. Put the cheese in it, thoroughly mixing it in.

10. Put the mixture into a 1.5 or 2-quart casserole dish.

11. Microwave or bake until hot.

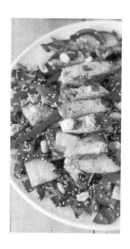

Ground Beef and Bell Peppers

Preparation time: 11 mins

Servings: 2

Nutritional Info: 380 Calories, 22g Fats, 6.2g Net Carbs, and 25g Protein.

Ingredients:

- 1 diced Onion
- Coconut oil
- 1 lb. beef, ground
- 1 c. freshly chopped Spinach
- Salt
- Pepper
- 1 sliced red Bell pepper

Directions:

1. Chop the spinach. Set aside.

2. Dice the onion into tiny pieces.

3. Add the oil to a skillet before placing the skillet on the stove over a burner set to a medium heat. Add in the onion and coat well in oil. Let it cook for 60 seconds.

4. Mix in the spinach and the beef and stir well. Season as desired.

5. Stir fry everything until cooked.

6. Put the sliced fresh bell pepper on a serving plate, and dish up the cooked meat mixture beside the peppers.

Snacks Recipes

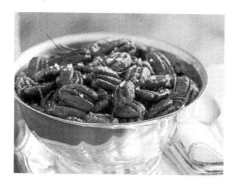

Brown-Butter Roasted Pecans with Rosemary

Preparation time: 20 mins

Servings: 4

Nutritional Information: 645 Calories, 66.6g Fats, 12.7g Net Carbs, and 9.2g Protein.

Ingredients:

- 4 c. pecan halves
- 2 tsps. sugar
- 2 tsps. kosher salt
- ¼ c. butter
- 1 tbsp. fresh rosemary, chopped
- Rosemary leaves, fresh

Directions:

1. Preheat the oven to 350F.

2. In a medium-sized saucepan; cook the butter over medium heat for about 3-5 minutes constantly stirring, until it starts to turn golden brown. Remove immediately from the heat; stir in the pecans. Arrange the butter coated pecans in a single layer on a baking sheet; sprinkle with the salt and sugar.

3. Bake pecans for about approximately 12 minutes, or until fragrant and toasted, stirring halfway through baking; sprinkle with the rosemary. Bake for another 2 minutes; let cool completely on the baking sheet, about 30 minutes.

4. Store in airtight container if there are any leftovers.

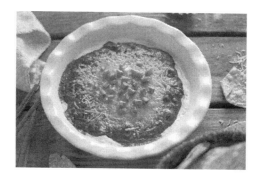

Cheesy Chili Dip

Preparation time: 10 mins

Servings: 8

Nutritional Information: 364 Calories, 31.9g Fats, 3.1g Net Carbs, and 16.9g Protein.

Ingredients:

- 10 ounces Kraft Old English cheese
- 4 ounces cream cheese
- ½ c. sour cream
- ¼ c. freshly chopped cilantro
- 2 tbsps. minced canned chipotle chili in adobo sauce

Directions:

1. In a food processor, blend the English cheese, cream cheese, sour cream, and chipotle until the mixture is soft. Stir in the cilantro, cover, and chill for at least 2 hours before serving.

2. Serve with assorted sliced vegetables or low carb chips or crackers.

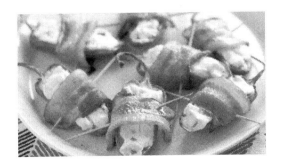

Bacon-Jalapeno Poppers

Preparation time: 15 mins

Servings: 12

Nutritional Information: 755 Calories, 61.7g Fats, 5.4g Net Carbs, and 43.2g Protein.

Ingredients:

- 25 jalapeno peppers, fresh
- 2 c. shredded cheddar cheese
- 16 oz. cream cheese
- 32 ounces chopped bacon

Directions:

1. Cut the stems of the jalapeño peppers and then cut them lengthwise; remove the seeds.

2. Fill each with the cream cheese; sprinkle the top with the cheddar cheese; and wrap each cheese-stuffed jalapeño with bacon.

3. Place on baking sheets, and bake for about 10-15 minutes in a 450F preheated oven, or until the bacon is cooked thoroughly.

4. Kill the heat and allow to cool; and serve.

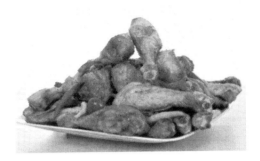

Oven-Fried Coconut Chicken Drumsticks

Preparation time: 10 mins

Servings: 4

Nutritional Information: 256 Calories, 8.6g Fats, 15.6g Net Carbs, and 27.7g Protein.

Ingredients:

- 2 large eggs
- 12 chicken drumsticks
- 1 c. coconut flour
- 1 c. shredded coconut, unsweetened
- 2 tbsps. coconut oil

Directions:

1. The first step is to preheat the oven to about 400 degrees Celsius
2. In a bowl, whisk the two eggs lightly
3. Mix the shredded coconut and the coconut flour in a bowl.

4. Each of the 12 drumsticks is dipped in the whisked egg then finally in the coconut mixture.

5. Place a pan in the oven to slightly heat before melting the 2 tablespoons of the coconut oil.

6. Fry each drumstick for about 2 minutes before placing them on a wire rack.

7. In an oven, place the wire rack containing the drumsticks for a minimum of 40 minutes.

8. After the 40 minutes, it is advisable to let the drumstick rest for a maximum of 10 minutes. This will allow the juices in the meat to settle.

9. The meal is ready for only 4 serves.

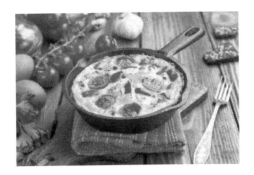

Three Cheese Bacon Tomato Frittata

Preparation time: 10 mins

Servings: 8

Nutritional Information: 210 Calories, 16.3g Fats, 2.9g Net Carbs, and 13.8g Protein.

Ingredients:

- 6 slices bacon
- 1 c. cherry tomatoes
- 10 large eggs
- ¼ c. heavy cream
- ¼ c. parmesan cheese
- ¼ c. feta cheese crumbles
- ½ c. sharp cheddar cheese, shredded

Directions:

1. First, it is important for you to slice the bacon to bite size. Fry the pieces over medium heat while on a pan. This is let until the bacon is crunchy.

2. Once the bacon has become crispy, add the sliced cherry tomatoes then cook for about 4 minutes.

3. Whisk all the 10 eggs in a large bowl. Add the ¼-cup cream into the bowl then mix them appropriately.

4. Include the cheese in the bowl containing the whisked eggs-cream mixture. Use a spatula to make a homogeneous mixture.

5. The ultimate egg mixture is poured in a pan then allowed to cook for like 2 minutes.

6. Into an oven with a temperature of about 375 degrees Celsius, place the pan containing the egg mixture for about 25 minutes.

7. The meal is ready to serve 8 dishes.

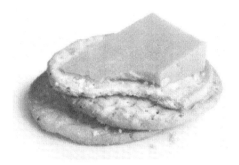

Sea Salt Cheese Crackers Gluten Free

Preparation time: 15 mins

Servings: 6

Nutritional Information: 130 Calories, 3g Fats, 22g Net Carbs, and 2g Protein.

Ingredients:

- 1 c. almond flour
- 1 large egg
- ¼ c. golden flax seed meal
- ½ tsp. baking soda
- Salt
- 1 c. sharp cheddar cheese

Directions:

1. In a food processor, add the almond flour, salt, baking soda, flax seed, and cheese. Turn on the processor to ensure the ingredients combine homogeneously.

2. To the uniform mixture, add oil and egg to form a ball.

3. Onto the cookie sheet, press the formed balls to make a dough

4. Sprinkle the salt over the dough. Using your hands spread the salt evenly over the whole area.

5. Use a pizza cutter to cut the flat almond mixture into smaller shapes of your choice.

6. Preheat the oven to about 350F for about 15 minutes.

7. While still hot, retrace the shapes you cut earlier using a pizza cutter.

8. Allow 10 minutes to cool the meal before enjoying the service.

9. Preheat outdoor grill on medium-high temperature, light oil the grate.

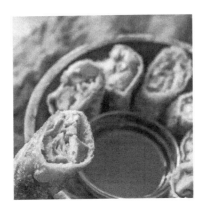

Avocado Slices

Preparation time: 5 mins

Servings: 2

Nutritional Information: 50 Calories, 5g Fats, 3g Net Carbs, and 1g Protein.

Ingredients:

- 2 ripe avocados
- ¼ c. coconut cream, whipped
- 1 c. almond meal
- 1 c. olive oil
- 1 cayenne pepper
- Salt

  Chili dip:

- 1 c. extra-virgin olive oil
- ½ c. almond milk

- 2 tsps. cider vinegar

- 1 tsp. chili powder

- Salt

Directions:

1. Peel, pit, and slice avocados.

2. Place whipped coconut cream in a small bowl.

3. In a separate bowl, combine almond meal with salt and cayenne pepper.

4. Heat oil in a deep pan.

5. Place avocado pieces into heated oil and fry 45 seconds.

6. Transfer to a paper-lined plate.

7. Make a chili dip; blend all dip ingredients, except the oil in a food blender until smooth. Stream in oil and blend until creamy. Serve with avocado slices.

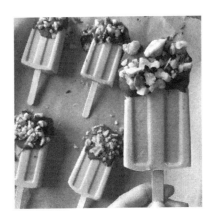

Icy Pops

Preparation time: 10 mins

Servings: 6

Nutritional Information: 41 Calories, 0.1g Fats, 10g Net Carbs, and 0g Protein.

Ingredients:

- 1 peeled and pitted avocado
- 1½ tsps. vanilla paste
- 1 c. coconut milk
- 2 tbsps. almond butter
- Drops of stevia
- ¼ tsp. Ceylon cinnamon

Directions:

1. Combine all ingredients in a food blender.
2. Blend until smooth.

3. Transfer the mixture into popsicle molds and insert popsicle sticks.

4. Freeze 4 hours or until firm.

5. Serve.

Desserts Recipes

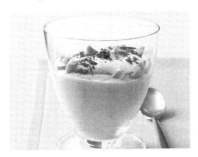

Peanut Butter Mousse

Preparation time: 2 mins

Servings: 4

Nutritional Information: 206 Calories, 18g Fats, 6g Net Carbs, and 5g Protein.

Ingredients:

- ½ can coconut cream
- 4 tablespoons natural peanut butter, unsweetened
- 1 teaspoon stevia

Directions:

1. Combine all ingredients and whip for one minute, until mixture forms peaks.
2. Chill for at least three hours, or until a mousse texture is achieved.

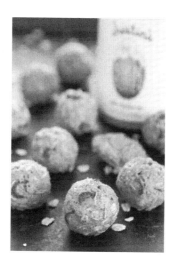

Almond butter balls

Preparation time: 10 mins

Servings: 14 balls

Nutritional Information: 135 Calories, 9g Fats, 18g Net Carbs, and 4g Protein.

Ingredients:

- 3 tbsps. almond butter
- 3 tbsps. carob powder
- 3 tsps. almond flour
- 2 tsps. powdered Yacon powder
- ½ c. coconut flakes, unsweetened

Directions:

1. In a bowl, combine almond butter, carob powder, almond flour, and Erythritol.

2. Stir until combined.

3. Place coconut flakes in a small bowl.

4. Scoop prepared a mixture with a small ice cream scoop and drop into coconut flakes.

5. Roll until completely covered with the coconut flakes. Arrange the balls on a plate and refrigerate for 4-6 hour or until firm.

6. Serve and enjoy.

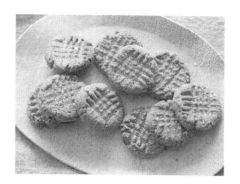

Peanut Butter Cookies

Preparation time: 10 mins

Servings: 12

Nutritional Information: 135 Calories, 7g Fats, 17g Net Carbs, and 2.6g Protein.

Ingredients:

- 1 c. smooth peanut butter
- ¾ c. almond flour
- ½ c. powdered Erythritol
- ¼ c. almond milk
- 1 scoop hemp protein powder, vanilla flavored
- 1 tsp. baking soda

Directions:

1. Heat oven to 350F and line a baking sheet with baking paper.

2. In a bowl, cream peanut butter, and powdered Erythritol.

3. In a separate bowl, combine all dry ingredients.

4. Fold the dry ingredients into peanut butter and stir until you have a crumbly mix.

5. Stir in almond milk and roll dough into balls (2 tablespoons per cookie).

6. Drop dough onto baking sheet and flatten with a fork, making a crisscross pattern.

7. Bake cookies 10 minutes. Cool completely before serving.

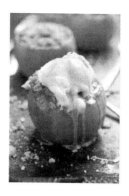

Stuffed Apples

Preparation time: 15 mins

Servings: 4

Nutritional Information: 352 Calories, 25.7g Fats, 34.5g Net Carbs, and 1.4g Protein.

Ingredients:

- 4 cored green apples
- ½ c. melted coconut butter
- ¼ c. almond butter, unsweetened
- 2 tbsps. Cinnamon, ground
- Ground nutmeg
- Salt
- 4 tbsps. Shredded and unsweetened coconut
- 1 c. water

Directions:

1. In a bowl, mix together coconut butter, almond butter, cinnamon, nutmeg and salt.

2. Arrange the apples in a slow cooker and place the water in the bottom. With a spoon, place butter mixture into each apple evenly. Top each apple with shredded coconut.

3. Set the slow cooker on Low. Cover and cook for about 2-3 hours.

4. Serve warm.

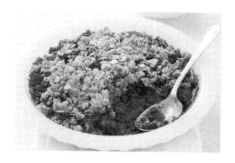

Berry Crumble

Preparation time: 20 mins

Servings: 6

Nutritional Information: 142 Calories, 10g Fats, 11.7g Net Carbs, and 1.9g Protein.

Ingredients:

- 1 c. almond flour
- 2 tbsps. melted butter
- 1 tbsp. applesauce, unsweetened
- 4 c. fresh mixed berries
- 1 tbsp. chopped butter

Directions:

1. In a bowl, add flour, melted butter and applesauce and mix until crumbly mixture forms.

2. In the bottom of a slow cooker, place the berries and dot with chopped butter. Sprinkle the topping mixture over the berries evenly.

3. Set the slow cooker on Low. Cover and cook for about 2 hours.

4. Unplug the slow cooker and let the crumble cool slightly. Cut into desired pieces and serve warm.

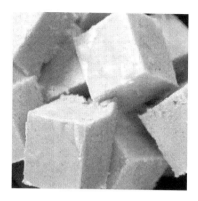

Cocoa Pumpkin Fudge

Preparation time: 10 mins

Servings: 24 slices

Nutritional Information: 91.1 Calories, 7.2g Fats, 8.5g Net Carbs, and 0.5g Protein.

Ingredients:

- 1 c. organic unsweetened pumpkin puree
- 1¾ c. cocoa butter
- 1 tsp. allspice
- 1 tbsp. coconut oil, melted

Directions:

1. Line 8-inch glass dish with baking paper.
2. Melt cocoa butter over medium heat.
3. Stir in pumpkin puree and allspice. Stir to combine.

4. Add coconut oil and stir well. Transfer the mixture into a prepared glass dish and press down to distribute evenly.

5. Cover with a second piece of baking paper and refrigerate 2 hours.

6. Slice and serve.

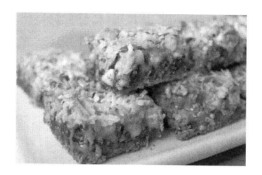

Coconut Cookie Bars

Preparation time: 10 mins

Servings: Makes 16 bars

Nutritional Information: 142 Calories, 14g Fats, 3g Net Carbs, and 2g Protein.

Ingredients:

- ¾ c. coconut butter

- ¼ c. apple sauce, unsweetened

- Salt

- 1¼ c. sesame seeds, raw

Directions:

1. Mix coconut butter, apple sauce, and salt until completely combined.

2. Add sesame seeds and stir together.

3. Bake in a greased muffin sheet at 350 degrees for 10 minutes, or until tops are brown.

4. Let them cool for 20 minutes before transferring to the freezer for 20 minutes to finish solidifying.

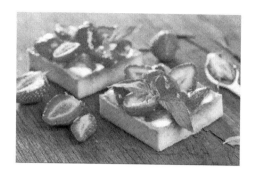

Keto Strawberry Shortcake

Preparation time: 30 mins

Servings: 1

Nutritional Information: 263 Calories, 24g Fats, 8g Net Carbs, and 7g Protein.

Ingredients:

- ½ tbsp. butter
- 2 tbsp. almond meal
- 1 c. chopped strawberries
- 1 tsp. vanilla syrup, sugar-free
- ½ c. cream

Directions:

1. Add the butter and the almond meal to a mug then place it in the oven for about 8-10 minutes. Preheat oven to 375 degrees F (190 C).

2. Use the spoon bottom to flatten the mixture and form a flat crust-like substance

3. Add the chopped blackberries into the mug containing the almond butter crust.

4. Blend the ½-cup heavy cream in a blender. This is the stage where you can add the sugar-free vanilla syrup as a sweetener.

5. Add the blended cream containing a sweetener (not a must) into the cup with the butter-almond meal combination.

6. For the crust to cool and be bread-like, place the mixture in the refrigerator for about 30 minutes.

7. After the timed a half an hour, the dessert is ready to be consumed as an after meal to meet your body desires.

Drinks

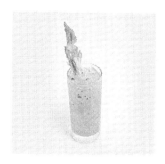

Celery Cup

Preparation time: 5 mins

Servings: 1

Nutritional Info: Calories 60, Total carbs 8g, Total Fats 0.7g, Protein 2g

Ingredients:

- 1 Celery
- ¼ C. cilantro
- 1 sliced cucumber
- 1 oz. lemon juice
- 1½ oz. Cucumber Vodka
- ¾ Agave

Directions:

1. Add everything to your shaker or blender and shake well, or pulse in your blender.

2. Pour into tall serving glass.

Red Snapper

Preparation time: 5 mins.

Serving: 1

Nutritional Info: Calories 40, Total Carbs 10g, Total fats 0g, Protein 2g

Ingredients:

- Red and yellow garden cherry tomatoes
- 2 oz. Gin
- ½ oz. lemon juice
- 5 shakes tobacco sauce
- 5 shakes Worcestershire sauce
- Salt
- Pepper

Directions:

1. Halve your smaller tomatoes and add everything into your shaker or a blender and pulse.

2. Pour into serving glass and serve.

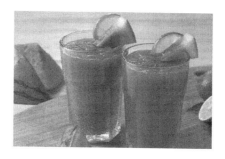

Watermelon Cooler

Preparation time: 5 mins

Servings: 2

Nutritional Info: Calories 150, Total Carbs 38g, Total Fats 0.1g, Protein 0g

Ingredients:

- 4 C seedless watermelon

- 1 C stemmed strawberries

- ½ lime, juice

- 2 tsp. chia seeds

Directions:

1. Add everything into your juicer and blend to pulp.

2. Discard any unwanted pulp and pour into two 8 oz. serving glasses.

3. Serve.

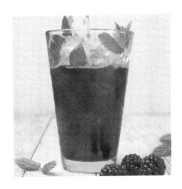

Blackberry Spritzer

Preparation time: 10 mins

Servings: 2

Nutritional Info: Calories 65, Total Carbs 14.7g, Total Fats 0.3g, Protein 2g

Ingredients:

- 1 2-liter spritzer soda
- ½ c. elderberry syrup
- 1 lone, juice
- 1/3 C. blackberries
- ¼ mint leaves, bruised

Directions:

1. Whisk the soda, syrup and lime.
2. Stir in the remaining ingredients.
3. Serve.

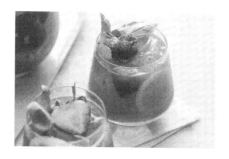

Strawberry Basil

Preparation time: 5 mins

Servings: 2

Nutritional Info: Calories 2, Total Fats 0g, Total Carbs 0.5g, Protein 0.1g

Ingredients:

- 1 lbs. strawberries, stemmed

- ½ juiced lemon

- ½ C packed basil leaves

- 1 C. sugar

- Carbonated Water

Directions:

1. Juice your strawberries in a juicer, according to juicer manufacturer's instructions, but you can go ahead and throw away the pulp.

2. Add strawberry juice into measuring glass, and water until you reach 1 C.

3. Pour the 1 C strawberry juice and water to saucepan and bring to a boil over medium heat.

4. Let simmer for about 5 minutes, and you want to make sure you are stirring the whole time.

5. Remove from heat, and strain the syrup, and get rid of any solid pieces, unless you like that.

6. Spoon 2 T syrup into your glass and add carbonated water, you can add syrup to your desired taste, store remaining syrup in fridge.

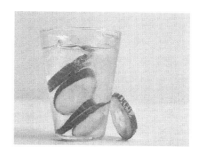

Cucumber Water

Preparation time: 5 mins

Servings: 4

Nutritional Info: Calories 0, Total Fats 0g, Total Carbs 0.5g, Protein 0.1g

Ingredients:

- 6-8 Cucumbers

Directions:

1. Peel the Cucumbers and chop.

2. Add the cucumber slices into your blender and pulp- about 1-2 minutes.

3. Place a strainer over bowl and pour juice into strainer from the blender.

4. Save Cucumber juice and drink, discard or repurpose the cucumber pulp.

5. Serve.

Conclusion

This is probably the best culinary trip you'll ever make! A Ketogenic diet is your chance to live a healthier and happier life! Trust us!Millions of people all over the world decide to start this diet each day and they all warmly recommend it!

A Ketogenic diet will soon show all its benefits and you will become a new person in no time!

In order to help you with this new lifestyle, we've decided to teach you how to prepare the best Ketogenic recipes!

That's why we developed this incredible cookbook! All you need to do is to take your time and discover each of our Ketogenic recipes!

It's going to be awesome! We guarantee it!

So, start a Ketogenic diet today and enjoy a new life!

Made in the USA
Middletown, DE
17 March 2018